MW01166659

Table of Contents

Menopause is a normal part of aging. As early as your 30s and 40s, your ovaries gradually start making smaller amounts of estrogen and progesterone. This is called "natural menopause." In the U.S., the average age when natural menopause occurs is 52 years old.

Some people experience menopause at a younger age. Early menopause is when your periods stop before age 45. Premature menopause is when they stop before age 40. Early menopause happens naturally in about 5% of women.

Causes of early and premature menopause include:

- Surgery to remove your ovaries (bilateral oophorectomy)
- Surgery to remove your uterus (hysterectomy)

- Chemotherapy and radiation treatment
- Family history of early or premature menopause
- Smoking
- Autoimmune conditions
- Other medical conditions

Menopause Symptoms

Menopause symptoms are the result of your reproductive hormone levels gradually decreasing in your body.

Two hormones, estrogen and progesterone, are especially important. These hormones are normally made by your ovaries, and help to control your menstrual cycle. And because these hormones have so many jobs in your body, they can cause many different types of symptoms.

With menopause, many people experience:

- Hot flashes and night sweats (in more than 80% of people)
- Sleep problems
- Vaginal thinning and loss of elasticity
- Vaginal dryness and irritation
- Dry skin, eyes, or mouth
- Frequent urinary tract infections (UTIs)
- Irritability
- Anxiety or low mood
- Poor concentration or "brain fog"
- Low libido
- Muscle and joint pain
- Fatigue

Symptoms can range from mild to severe, and can happen before, during, and even after menopause.

Some people even feel better, because they're not dealing with regular periods.

Menopause Diagnosis

Am I in menopause?

There's no simple test that can confirm whether you are in menopause. Most people are able to tell they are going through menopause on the basis of their age and symptoms. And if you've gone 12 months or more without a period (without another cause), you may have already completed menopause.

When to see a doctor

For most people, menopause is a natural part of aging. You do not need medical treatment to go through menopause. But if you are having menopause symptoms especially if they are bothersome you may want to consider talking to your healthcare provider.

Depending on your age and medical history, your healthcare provider may suggest blood tests to check your hormone levels — and to rule out other causes for your symptoms, like thyroid problems. These tests may include checking your levels of:

- Follicle-stimulating hormone (FSH)
- Estrogen (estradiol)
- Thyroid-stimulating hormone (TSH)

Finally, you should always see a provider if you have bleeding from your vagina after menopause. Postmenopausal bleeding can be an early warning sign of a serious health condition, like uterine cancer.

Medications

Hormone replacement therapy (HRT) is the most effective overall treatment for menopause symptoms. HRT can help with body-wide symptoms like:

- Hot flashes
- Night sweats
- Mood changes
- Vaginal dryness
- Bone loss and fragility

HRT replaces the hormones that your ovaries were making before menopause. It's generally considered safe if you start before age 60, or within 10 years of completing menopause.

Other prescription medications can also help:

Low-dose antidepressants: Low doses of certain antidepressants can help with hot flashes. These medications can also be used at higher doses to help with mood or anxiety.

Gabapentin: This is an anti-seizure medication that can reduce hot flashes. In some cases, it can also be used for mood or anxiety.

Clonidine: Clonidine is a blood-pressure medication that can help with hot flashes.

Osteoporosis medications: These are medications that help reduce bone loss and protect you from fractures.

Menopause Treatments

There are many non-medication treatments that can help support you during menopause and beyond. In fact, 50% of people use natural treatments during menopause. Examples include:

- Phytoestrogen foods or supplements: Phytoestrogens are plant compounds that have estrogen-like effects in your body. Phytoestrogens are found in many different foods and supplements, including soy, flaxseed, and red clover.
- Calcium and vitamin D: These do not directly help with menopause symptoms, but can support strong bones and decrease your risk of osteoporosis.
- Herbal supplements: There are many different supplements marketed for use during menopause. Read more in our guide to natural treatments.
- Diet and lifestyle changes: Sleep, exercise, eating well, and cutting down on smoking can

all help with menopause symptoms. These changes can also protect your bones and heart, and support your long-term health.

- Mind–body treatments: Acupuncture, hypnosis, and mindfulness-based stress reduction can all potentially have benefits during menopause.

Living

Though menopause is a natural part of getting older, it can still affect your overall health. It's important to keep up with preventive care during and after menopause, by seeing your provider regularly for a wellness exam.

During and after menopause it's especially important to take care of your:

- Heart and blood vessels: Protect yourself from heart disease by eating heart-healthy foods, exercising, and maintaining a healthy body weight.

- Bones: Support healthy bones by eating a calcium-rich diet, getting enough vitamin D, and exercising.

- Pelvic muscles: Kegel exercises can strengthen the muscles in your genital area and pelvic floor. Surgery or special devices can also help in some cases.

- Sexual health: Water- or silicone-based lubricants and moisturizers can help with comfort and pleasure.

- Weight: Many people gain weight after menopause. If weight is a concern, consider adding more physical movement into your daily life, or reducing your daily calorie intake.

Broadly speaking, there are two different kinds of sleep disturbances, says Dr. Monica Christmas, Assistant Professor of Obstetrics and Gynecology at the University of Chicago Medical School. One is caused by night sweats, in which case, "managing the night sweats will take care of the sleep quality."

This can be addressed with hormone therapy, as well as some SSRIs (selective serotonin reuptake inhibitors) and other psych meds that have recently been found to reduce vasomotor symptoms such as hot flashes and night sweats, though there are other less medical approaches you can try to make yourself more comfortable as well.

If night sweats are not the only thing causing the changes in your sleep uality, Dr. Christmas highly recommends cognitive behavioral therapy (CBT). "CBT techniques have been shown to be helpful," she says, noting that even if you don't have access to a sleep therapist, there are apps and other resources that teach you tricks for better sleep. Mindfulness can be extremely helpful, and that doesn't have to mean actual meditation, it's more about learning how to calm and self soothe yourself through a sleepless night.

Tips for Getting a Better Night's Sleep During Menopause

Banish anything electric that stimulates your brain.

Don't use your phone as an alarm clock or look at it right before bed.

Keep your room cool and dark.

If you do wake, get up and read a book. "That actually tends to fatigue us again," Dr. Christmas says.

Watch your food and drink triggers before bed. Try reducing how often and how much alcohol you drink at night, in addition to any caffeinated beverages.

Do some regular exercise earlier in the day, especially weight-bearing exercise or yoga. We start losing muscle mass and bone mass at this time, and weight-bearing exercises (including walking) have been shown to counteract both as well as reduce vaginal symptoms, as they engage your core and pelvic floor.

Proactively manage any anxiety and depression, and seek mental health help if you are not feeling like yourself emotionally.

If you are experiencing any other symptoms as well, this kind of sleep disturbance might still be helped with hormone therapy, especially as progesterone aids in sleep.

How to Handle Hot Flashes During Menopause

Hormone therapy is the most effective tool. If you can't take hormone therapy, don't despair. There are more treatments for vasomotor symptoms than ever before, including the many SSRIs and anti-anxiety meds that have been found to have the welcome bonus of reducing hot flashes, making them a good option if you are having emotional and mental health symptoms along with your physical ones.

That said, many lifestyle interventions will also help, especially in combination, including:

Cognitive behavioral therapy (CBT)

As with sleep, yoga has been found to relieve hot flashes.

Exercise

If you are a smoker, one of the most important things you can do for your health is to stop smoking. It's linked with earlier perimenopause. But, once you're in perimenopause, stopping can also help minimize the severity of hot flashes during menopause and beyond.

You may also want to start limiting alcohol. We all become more sensitive to its effects as we grow older, and the associated health risks rise. Research seems to show that once you're postmenopause, drinking can trigger hot flashes.

What to Do About Vaginal Symptoms During Menopause

For vaginal dryness during sex or that's bothering you any other time, there are a wide array of lubes and vaginal moisturizers to choose from. Products such as Revaree, Good Clean Love and Ah Yes! are made without fragrance and tend to be closer to the consistency of natural vaginal secretions think slippery and liquid as opposed to sticky and viscous.

You can use a vaginal moisturizer the same way you would any other type of moisturizer, daily or as needed, and women tend to have personal preferences toward which one they like the same way they do for facial moisturizer.

If you feel like OTC products just aren't cutting it, there are also plenty of estrogen creams, gels, suppositories, and even a vaginal ring that slowly releases a low dose of estrogen to choose from. If your menopausal symptoms are mostly around your vagina, localized estrogen, no matter what method you prefer, is one way to take a lower dose of hormone therapy that is only targeting that specific area as opposed to affecting your whole body.

As with birth control and contraceptive hormones, different women tend to have different hormone therapy delivery methods they prefer during menopause, and it may take you some trial and error with the help of your NAMS-certified menopause practitioner to arrive at the method and dose of hormone therapy that feels best for you. Or you may not want to try HT at all, and that's perfectly fine too.

For Overactive Bladder (OAB), Try Giving Your Pelvic Floor Some Attention

This is a group of muscles supporting your core and abdominal organs. Over time it can become weak or stressed, particularly after childbirth, leading to issues like incontinence that can progress with age. Doing Kegel exercises can help. Now is a good time to see a pelvic floor specialist who can evaluate you and teach you how to do those Kegels effectively. In popular culture, Kegels tend to be discussed as a simple clenching and unclenching, but when done correctly, they are more like slowly pulling an imaginary ball up a long hallway and then slowly releasing it back down. Pilates is also a form of exercise that specifically targets your pelvic floor, so it's worth giving it a try as you enter perimenopause if you feel like your pelvic floor could use a little TLC.

What Is Hormone Therapy?

Can you take more estrogen and progesterone to return yourself back to "normal?" Not exactly, but you can get hormone therapy (HT) to help make yourself more comfortable if you have been feeling uncomfortable or irritable and to help lower your risk for diseases like osteoporosis which are linked to less estrogen.

It used to be called hormone replacement therapy, but the name has changed because the goal isn't to "replace" the estrogen to premenopausal levels, but to provide the minimal amount needed to relieve hot flashes and other menopausal conditions if and when they're bothering you. Let's take a look at some of the hormone therapies available today.

Estrogen-Progestogen Therapy

Most menopausal women who do hormone therapy use a combination of estrogen and progestogen. This is because when taken alone, estrogen can increase your risk for certain types of cancer, which progesterone can help to mitigate.

Estrogen therapy comes in two main types. "Systemic" delivers estrogen throughout your body and can come as a patch you place directly on your skin or as a tablet. "Local" delivers a low dose of estrogen directly to your vagina to address vaginal symptoms and can come as a cream, gel, or an inserted ring.

Progestogen therapy can come in the form of natural progesterone or synthetic progestin, as well as an IUD.

With long term use (more than 5 years), there is an increased risk of breast cancer, blood clots, and stroke. Because of the breast cancer risk, many doctors do not recommend estrogen-progestogen therapy for women with a family history of breast cancer (they occasionally prescribe progestogen-only, which can provide some relief for hot flashes and sleep issues). This is also why the menopause mantra for HT that you will hear repeatedly is to take the lowest dose for the shortest time that is effective to treat your symptoms.

If you are not eligible for hormone therapy, don't despair. There are more non-hormonal menopause treatments than ever before, including SSRIs, anti-anxiety meds, steroids, and other medications that have recently been found to also relieve menopausal symptoms, so make sure to check with your NCMP to find the solution that's best for you, no matter what your reasons are for being unable to try hormone therapy.

How Do You Decide If Hormone Therapy Is Right for You?

It depends on what your goals are. Here are a few uestions to consider.

What are you trying to treat? If you want to relieve hot flashes, night sweats and related sleep disturbances, manage mood swings, reduce urinary incontinence; and prevent bone loss, HT can help.

How intense are those symptoms? How much do they disrupt your life?

Are there any contraindications? For example, do you have undiagnosed vaginal bleeding, breast or uterine cancer, a history of blood clots, heart attack, or stroke risk?

What is your age and how far past menopause (if at all) are you? The risks and outcomes look better for people who start HT under the age of 60 and as soon as possible in relation to when they first enter menopause. (Beyond that, the risk for heart disease, stroke, and dementia rise.) This is why the recommendation is to start HT at the first signs of bothersome menopause symptoms at the lowest dose for the shortest possible time.

Hormone therapy delivers major relief for a lot of people, and for many, it is by far the most effective menopause treatment. But its intended purpose isn't to turn back time and return you back to "normal," whatever that means.

The menopause train has left the station and you are on this ride no matter what. HT is not going to make everything all better either. For best results with HT, getting your lifestyle on the right track (nutrition, movement, sleep habits, mental health) will drastically help improve its efficacy.

How Safe Is Hormone Therapy?

Women enjoyed the benefits of HT from the 1970s until 2002, when the bottom fell out. That's the year the Women's Health Initiative (WHI) trial released its findings. The study focused on 16,600 American women aged 50-79. Half of those women were randomly selected to take oral estrogen combined with progesterone HT for 5 years and the other half took a placebo.

The trial found that the women on HT were at increased risk for breast cancer, heart disease, stroke, blood clots, and urinary incontinence. Alarmed by media reports, doctors stopped prescribing HT and women stopped asking for it. As a result, the prevalence of use dropped from 19% in 2000 to 4.9% by 2009. The trial found that the women on HT were at increased risk for breast cancer, heart disease, stroke, blood clots, and urinary incontinence. Alarmed by media reports, doctors stopped prescribing HT and women stopped asking for it. As a result, the prevalence of use dropped from 19% in 2000 to 4.9% by 2009).

However, further analysis of the study later found nuances that had been lost in the initial report. Namely, HT was actually health-protective for women under 60 (a third of the women in the study), while it was the women who started HT after 70 who faced greater health risks than benefits.

Also, the study looked at one combined dose only, a dose considered appropriate for women over 60 but too high for women in their 70s, and higher than the dose most women use today. We know now that if you start at the lowest dose earlier instead of a high dose later, risks decrease, and health-protective effects increase.

5 Reasons Why Some Women Go Through Early Menopause

Maybe you wake up at night drenched in sweat. Or you're struggling to concentrate, and oh yeah, your period has been MIA. These symptoms are enough to freak any woman out, even when she's at the right age for menopause, the natural transition to infertility that most women experience around 50. But when these symptoms begin in your 30s, they can be downright scary.

For some women, early menopause is brought on by surgery that removes the ovaries. A woman who carries a BRCA gene mutation, for example, may opt to have her ovaries and fallopian tubes taken out in a preventative salpingo-oopherectomy. (This is the procedure Angelina Jolie, after blood tests revealed possible indicators of early cancer.) The result? Levels of estrogen and other female hormones drop dramatically, which may lead to hot flashes, vaginal dryness, and other telltale signs of menopause.

But one in 100 women will experience these symptoms by the age of 40 for other reasons—which are often hard to pin down. In fact, in about 90 percent of cases, a woman never learns the reason why. The technical term for this medical condition is primary ovarian insufficiency (POI). "Basically the ovaries poop out early," explains Shawn Tassone, MD, an OB-GYN who specializes in integrative medicine at Austin Area Obstetrics, Gynecology, and Fertility.

One key sign for diagnosis: skipped or irregular periods for four months. Women with POI (also known as premature ovarian failure) may face more than mood swings and low libido. If they want to have children, they will likely struggle with infertility, and that can be the first sign that something is not right.

(That said, some women do continue to have occasional periods for years after a POI diagnosis, and between 5 percent and 10 percent do manage to get pregnant.)

Although most of the time POI happens without an obvious cause, there are quite a few things that are known to bring it on—yet many women are unaware of them. Below are the top factors that put you at risk.

Your Mom Went Through Early Menopause

Or your sister, or your grandmother. POI seems to be genetic: "You tend to see it run in families," Dr. Tassone says. "It can come from either side." A 2011 review of studies found that in up to 20 percent of cases, the woman has a family history of the condition.

Genetic Disorders

FMR1 is a gene that causes Fragile X syndrome, the most common form of inherited intellectual impairment; even if you don't have the syndrome you can have a mutation on that same gene that causes problems with your ovaries, leading to fragile X-associated primary ovarian insufficiency. According to a report by the National Institutes of Health, this is the case for one in 33 women with POI.

Turner Syndrome (in which a woman has only one X chromosome) is another genetic disorder associated with POI.

Autoimmune Disorders

The autoimmune disorder thyroiditis (inflammation of the thyroid gland) has been linked to POI. So has Addison's Disease, in which the adrenal glands don't produce enough hormones. In the case of either of these diseases, it's possible your own immune system may begin to attack the follicles in your ovaries, the small sacs where eggs mature and grow, interfering with their ability to function.

Smoking or Other Toxin Exposure

"Some toxins can bring on premature ovarian failure," Dr. Tassone says. "Things like cigarettes and pesticides." Normally we are born with enough primordial follicles (aka the tiny seeds that grow into follicles) to last us until the natural age of menopause, around 50. But exposure to harmful chemicals is thought to cause a woman to run out of follicles sooner rather than later.

Chemotherapy or Radiation

Similar to environmental toxins, these cancer treatments can damage the genetic material in ovarian cells. But the damage depends on various factors, like the type of drug and dose of radiation, your age at the time of treatment, and the area of your body that was radiated. Some women may not develop POI until years after undergoing cancer treatment. And some won't ever get it.

What are the Best Foods to Eat During the Menopause and Beyond?

The menopause can be a difficult time for many women and so it is very understandable why many are drawn to the idea of supplements or changing their diet to help. But is there any evidence to back any of the claims? Can anything help with symptoms? Can changes you make to your diet help with your long-term health?

This books talks through the evidence behind supplements, dietary changes for menopausal symptoms, and how to reduce both your long-term risk of cardiovascular disease and osteoporosis.

Dietary Changes for Menopausal Symptoms

Caffeine and Alcohol

Reducing caffeine, alcohol and spicy food in your diet may help hot flushes, but there is considerable variation between individuals Current recommended limits of alcohol are a total of 14 units a week, with a maximum of two per day. Reducing alcohol also has other health benefits, such as a lower risk of liver disease, heart disease, osteoporosis, type 2 diabetes, and certain types of cancer such as breast cancer.

Magnesium Supplements

For some women insomnia can be a symptom of the menopause. Unfortunately, there is very little evidence to support any benefit from magnesium supplements. Instead you should be able to meet all your magnesium needs through a healthy diet containing wholegrains, spinach, pumpkin seeds, almonds and beans.

Phytoestrogens

Phytoestrogens are plant derived compounds, that have a similar structure to human estrogen, and similar but weaker activity. They are found in foods and in a more concentrated form in supplements.

Phytoestrogens supplements are fre uently marketed and chosen to target hot flushes.

Herbal Medicines That Contain Phytoestrogens

There are a number of herbal medicines that contain phytoestrogens that may help with the symptoms of menopause. There is evidence to support decreased hot flushes with St John's wort, black cohosh and genistein.

Isoflavones (soya products and red clover) are a type of phytoestrogen. There is mixed evidence that they may reduce hot flushes. Red clover is not advised in women with breast cancer, but soya is probably safe. These supplements may also interact with other medications such as those for heart disease, epilepsy and asthma, so you should speak with your GP before starting any herbal medicine.

The contents of herbal medicines may vary considerably, as in contrast to conventional medicine, there is no legal obligation for herbal medicines to be licenced. Check for a product licence or Traditional Herbal Registration (THR) number on the label and always buy from a reputable setting.

Foods That Contain Phytoestrogens

The phytoestrogens found naturally in some foods are less concentrated than supplements. Phytoestrogens occur naturally in some plant-based foods such as:

- Soybeans and soy based products
- Peanuts
- Sesame seeds
- Flaxseeds
- Chickpeas
- Berries

- Barley
- Apricots
- Tea (green and black)

Given the mixed evidence about efficacy of the supplements, is therefore unlikely that consuming these food items, will have a significant benefit on symptoms.

Dietary Changes for Long Term-Health

Declining levels of estrogen from the menopause and beyond increases your risk of cardiovascular disease (heart disease and strokes) and osteoporosis (brittle bones and increased risk of fractures), diabetes, depression, obesity and dementia. If you experience early or premature menopause, your risk is unfortunately higher. To counteract these concerns you can make some dietary changes to reduce your long-term risks.

Optimising Bone Health

Osteoporosis leads to a greater risk of having low energy fractures. Estrogen has a really important role in bone health, and as levels decline, risk of osteoporosis increases. A 50 year old woman only has a 2% risk of osteoporosis, compared with a 25% risk in an 80 year old lady, due to considerably lower levels of estrogen.

Diet can play an important role in bone health. There are some key macronutrients, vitamins and minerals to be sure that you are getting enough of:

Quality protein: Include lean protein foods at every meal such as seafood, beans, legumes, dairy, meat, and poultry.

Calcium is an important mineral for bone health, and as an adult before the menopause you need to 700mg per day while from the menopause this rises to 1200mg a day. Good sources of calcium include dairy, calcium-fortified plant-based drinks, tinned fish (with bones), spinach, fortified bread, baked beans, tofu and dried figs. If you are unable to have enough in your diet, you might be prescribed a supplement.

Vitamin D, commonly called the sunshine vitamin as it is produced by the action of sunlight on our skin during exposure outside. Current NHS guidance is for women to consider taking a supplement of 10mcg (400IU) during the autumn and winter months as it can be difficult to get enough sun exposure. Vitamin D is also found in low levels egg yolks, oily fish and some fortified foods, but is difficult to get enough from diet alone. It was previously thought that sunscreen prevented vitamin D formation, but evidence suggests that sunscreen does not inhibit vitamin D production in the skin.

The term vitamin K covers a number of different molecules and you need to eat a range of items to ensure you get all the different elements. Vitamin K is found in green vegetables, fermented food, dairy, and meat and has an important role in bone strength. Although there is mixed evidence as to whether vitamin K supplementation improves bone strength and reduces fractures, a number of countries for example Japan, now include vitamin K supplementation as treatment for osteoporosis. Vitamin K is a fat-soluble vitamin, and is stored if you take excess. It is therefore possible to have too much through supplementation, and we don't know what these effects might be. If you are on blood thinning medication, you should avoid taking vitamin K supplements as they can interfere.

Phosphorus is found in foods such as poultry, meat, dairy, oily fish, potatoes, wholegrains, pulses and beans. It is usually abundant in our diet, and you should not need to take a supplement.

Magnesium is another mineral that is usually abundant in our diet but good sources include wholegrains, spinach, pumpkin seeds, almonds and beans. Again you should not need to supplement this.

Resistance exercise is very important for bone strength. The NHS advise 30 minutes twice a week for adults over the age of 35 years. Examples include brisk walking, resistance bands, yoga, squats, weight training, Pilates, gardening and a brisk walk.

Reducing Risk of Cardiovascular Disease (CVD)

The risk of cardiovascular disease increases during and after the menopause. This is partly related to the aging process, and also the effects of declining estrogen. Cardiovascular disease is a general term used for conditions affecting blood vessels and the heart by narrowing of the arteries (atherosclerosis) and an increased risk of blood clots such as strokes.

Weight gain associated with declining estrogen levels also leads to an increased risk of obesity, higher blood pressure, type 2 diabetes, and higher (LDL) cholesterol levels, which are all well recognised as factors for CVD

There is evidence that dietary changes can help reduce this risk so aim to follow a diet with the following principles:

- Swap saturated fats (animal fats) to unsaturated fats such as extra virgin olive oil, rapeseed oil, avocado, seeds, nuts
- Reduce fat content to less than 30% of your diet (approximately 60g per day)
- Swap refined carbohydrates (white bread, white rice) with whole-grains (brown rice, brown bread, millet, teff, bulgur wheat).
- Eat at least 5 portions of fruit and vegetables a day
- Aim to have 2 portions of oily fish (for example salmon, sardines, mackerel) twice a week. If you do not eat fish, have daily nuts, and seeds which also contain omega 3.
- Aim for a handful of nuts and seeds a day.
- Regularly enjoy beans, lentils and chickpeas.
- Avoid convenience products that have high amounts of sugar and salt, and sugary fizzy drinks.

- Try to reduce alcohol, and try to keep less than 14 units of alcohol per week (maximum of 2 units per day).

Maintaining a Healthy Weight

A healthy weight can help reduce your risk of diabetes and cardiovascular disease, however this can be harder with declining levels of estrogen. To understand the role estrogen plays, it helps to understand about metabolism and basal metabolic rate first.

Metabolism is the production of energy from food, whereas the basal metabolic rate (BMR) is the energy re uired for performing vital body functions at complete rest or asleep. Our brain, liver, heart and kidneys account for almost half of the BMR. An estimate of BMR can be calculated from weight, age and gender. Our BMR accounts for most of the energy we use, with thermogenesis only 10% and physical activity between 10-30%.

Your basal metabolic rate is determined by your genes, your body composition and your sex hormones. Exercise can increase your BMR and is important for so many factors of general health.

What is the Role of Estrogen in Energy Balance and Metabolism?

The main circulating form of estrogen in the body is 17β-estradiol (E2). E2 promotes energy homeostasis, improves body fat distribution, enhances insulin sensitivity, improves pancreatic β-cell function, and reduces inflammation. As estrogen levels naturally decline from perimenopause, there is an increased risk of developing metabolic dysfunction, leading to obesity, the metabolic syndrome, type 2 diabetes as well as cancers and other degenerative diseases of the skeletal, central nervous and cardiovascular systems. This role in energy metabolism is also supported by findings in evolutionary development (phylogeny) since ancestral estrogen receptors have been found in invertebrates before advent of sexual reproduction.

Estrogen also has a role in energy balance, acting in the hypothalamic area of the brain to both suppresses food intake and also stimulate physical activity, energy expenditure and regulate body fat distribution. The BMR varies across the menstrual cycle, and is lowest in the follicular phase (from the start of your period to ovulation), when ovarian hormones are lowest. Experiments on rodents have found that surgical removal of the ovaries leads to weight gain, which is reversed by estrogen supplements.

In summary, estrogen has an important role in energy balance, BMR and weight gain. As levels naturally decline at the perimenopause, increasing weight is linked with increased risk of cardiovascular disease and diabetes.

BMR is determined by our genes, our body composition and our sex hormones. Exercise can increase BMR and is important for so many factors of general health. While maintaining a steady weight used to be thought of in terms of simple energy balance, evidence of the important role of the gut microbiota, might explain why some people can appear to eat much more than the energy they expend, without gaining weight.

Microbiota and Their Role in Metabolism

The gut microbiota contains trillions of single celled microorganisms, that play an important role in our health. Multiple associations between the gut microbiota and chemicals along metabolic pathways have been found, with suggestion that the gut microorganisms have a role in shaping metabolism. Recent research has found that changing the composition of the microbiota, is associated with improvement of some of the parameters of the metabolic syndrome (a name given to a set of conditions seen together including increased blood pressure, high blood sugar, a large waistline, and abnormal cholesterol or triglyceride levels).

In studies of special germ-free mice, who have no organisms living on or inside them, they found that faecal transplant from obese humans, was associated with a greater weight gain than mice that received microbes from healthy weight humans. This suggests that maintenance of a steady healthy weight, is more than the simple balance of energy in, equalling energy out. Instead, it is also impacted by your gut microbiota. Most studies of people that were obese have found that their gut microbiota is characterised by a narrower range of organisms (lower diversity). Long term weight gain (over 10 years) in humans is correlated with low microbiota diversity (narrow range of species of microorganisms), and this association is worsened by low dietary fibre intake.

How single celled microorganisms have such a profound effect on our weight and general health is astonishing, but it is probably mediated by a number of different routes. Gut microbiota imbalance probably promotes weight gain and metabolic complications by a variety of mechanisms including immune dysregulation, altered energy regulation, altered gut hormone regulation, and proinflammatory mechanisms (such as lipopolysaccharide endotoxins crossing the gut barrier and entering the portal circulation)

The menopause is a time of immense change, with women experiencing a spectrum of severity of symptoms. Dietary changes might not be possible for you right away, but try to incorporate them where possible for long-term health benefits.

Aim to eat a variety of colours, whole grains, quality protein at every meal, unsaturated fats, whole plant-based foods, items rich in calcium and optimise your gut health.

Ultimately the best way to support a healthy weight, reduced long-term risk of cardiovascular disease and osteoporosis is by regular exercise and a healthy diet that follows these principles:

- Eat lots of different coloured fruit and vegetables.
- Choose wholegrains (bulgur wheat, millet, sweet potatoes, brown rice, brown bread).
- Eat a handful of nuts a day and add seeds to your food.
- Eat oily fish twice a week. If you do not eat fish, have daily nuts, and seeds which also contain omega 3.
- Chose lean or plant-based protein at every meal.
- Regularly enjoy beans, lentils and chickpeas.
- Enjoy healthy unsaturated fats such avocados, rapeseed, nuts and extra virgin olive oils.
- Aim for a handful of nuts and seeds a day.
- Avoid convenience products that have high amounts of sugar and salt, and sugary fizzy drinks.

- Avoid sweeteners.
- Support your microbiota to flourish by eating fermented foods, kefir, and 30g of fibre a day.
- Try to reduce alcohol, and try to keep less than 14 units of alcohol per week (maximum of 2 units per day).
- Enjoy lots of calcium rich foods (1200mg per day from the menopause onwards).

1. Banana muffins

Ingredients

100g plain wholemeal flour

25g soya flour

3 tablespoons light muscovado sugar

2 teaspoons baking powder

1 egg, beaten

50 ml soya milk

50ml sunflower oil

2 ripe bananas, about 200g when peeled and mashed

Topping:

1 tablespoon golden linseeds

25g self-raising flour, sifted

15g butter (room temperature)

40g Demerara sugar

1/2 teaspoon ground cinnamon

1 tablespoon water

Method

Grease 6 muffin tins or line with paper muffin cases

Pre heat oven to 200C/400F/Gas mark 6

To make muffins:

Place the wholemeal and soya flours, sugar, baking powder in a bowl, mix together. Make a well in the centre.

In a separate bowl, mix the egg, soya milk and oil together. Pour the li uid in to the flour. Stir until just blended. Gently stir in the bananas.

To make the topping:

Place the linseeds In a blender or food processor for 30 seconds.

Place the self-raising flour in a bowl and rub in the butter until the mixture is like fine breadcrumbs. Add the Demerara sugar, linseeds and cinnamon, then stir in the water and mix well.

Fill the muffin tins or cases two-thirds full of muffin mixture, then sprinkle topping over each muffin.

Place in the oven for 25-30 minutes.

Transfer to a wire rack to cool.

2. **Fresh fruit salad with linseeds and soya yoghurt**

Ingredients

200g seedless grapes

2 bananas

2 pears

2 apples

2 oranges

200g of fruit in season such as strawberries, blueberries, melon

2 tablespoons linseeds

4 tablespoons honey

2 tablespoons hot water

Serve with soya yoghurt

Method

Mix the honey with the warm water in a large bowl. Prepare the fruit and add to the bowl including any juices.

Add berries and soya yoghurt just before serving.

3. Home made granola

Ingredients

300g rolled oats

50g sunflower seeds

4 tbsp sesame seeds

4 tbsp linseeds

50g pumpkin seeds

50g flaked almonds

50g roasted hazelnuts

100g dried cranberries or cherries

50g unsweetened desiccated coconut

100ml maple syrup

2 tbsp honey

2 tbsp rapeseed oil

Directions

Heat the oven to 300F/150C/Gas 2.

Mix the oil, honey, maple syrup together in a large bowl. Add the seeds, the almonds and hazelnuts and mix well. Tip the mixture on to two baking sheets and spread evenly. Bake for 10-12 minutes. Add the coconut and dried fruit and bake for a further 15 minutes. Remove from the oven and scrape on to a flat tray to cool.

Serve with soya milk, almond milk or yoghurt and fresh fruit such as berries or grated apple. The granola can be stored in an airtight container for up to one month.

4. Miso soup

Ingredients

225g tofu

400ml water

2 tablespoons miso

2 spring onions, finely chopped

10g dried wakame

Directions

Soak the wakame in a large bowl of cold water for 10 minutes. Drain. Chop in to small 1cm pieces.

Cut tofu in to 1 cm s uares.

Boil the water in a saucepan. In a separate cup, add 3 tablespoons of hot water to the miso, then add to the saucepan. Add the wakame and the tofu and bring almost to the boil again. Add the spring onions. Remove from the heat and serve.

5. Minestrone soup

Ingredients

1.5 litres of miso soup or vegetable stock

200g tomatoes, skinned and roughly chopped

175g new potatoes, sliced

175g spring cabbage, shredded finely

175g small carrots, sliced

175g courgettes, chopped

175g green beans cut into 1 cm pieces

50g fresh peas, shelled

4 tender celery sticks, finely sliced

2 leeks, thinly sliced

1 large onion, finely chopped

1 clove garlic, chopped

1 bay leaf

2 tablespoons olive oil

8 fresh basil leave sprigs

85g soup pasta, such as vermicelli

50g borlotti beans

50g dried cannellini beans

Sea salt and black pepper

Garlic croutons to serve

Directions

Soak the beans in water for a few hours than drain and rinse.

Heat the olive oil in a big saucepan, then add the onion, garlic and bay leaf and sauté for about 4 minutes. Add the carrots, celery and leeks and cook for 4 minutes. Add the drained beans and sauté for another 4 minutes. Add the courgettes, green beans and peas and sauté for another 4 minutes. Add the water, miso soup or vegetable stock with the tomatoes, cabbage and potatoes and bring to the boil. Cover and simmer gently for 90 minutes until the beans are tender. Season to taste. Add in the pasta and basil and cook for a further 15 minutes until the pasta is cooked. Serve with garlic croutons.

6. Mixed bean casserole soup

Ingredients

1.5 litres vegetable stock, hot

225g cabbage, shredded

225g green beans, chopped

225g potatoes, chopped

8 sprigs of basil

4 basil leaves, for garnish

4 garlic cloves

2 carrots, chopped

1 onion, chopped

6 tablespoons olive oil

4 tablespoons freshly grated parmesan cheese

150g dried haricot beans, soaked for several hours

150g dried flageolet beans, soaked for several hours

Directions

Heat the oven to 220C/400F/Gas 6

Drain the soaked beans and put them in a large casserole dish, cover with 6cm of water. Add the onions. Cover and cook in the oven for 11/2 hours. Drain. Take half the beans and onion mixture and puree. Return the beans and bean puree to the casserole dish. Add the hot vegetable stock, the carrots, cabbage, potato and green beans. Season with salt and pepper. Cover and put in the oven at slightly lower temperature 180/350/gas 4 and cook for 45-60 minutes until the vegetables are tender. Meanwhile in a separate dish, crush the garlic and 8 basil sprigs and gradually add the olive oil. Then add the parmesan. Stir half this mixture in to the soup just before serving and then pour the soup in to bowls. Top each bowl of soup with a dessert spoonful of the garlic, basil oil and parmesan mixture. Garnish soup with basil.

7. Fruity rice salad

Ingredients

120g brown rice

225g tin of pineapple pieces, in juice

225g sweetcorn

50g sultanas

Small red pepper, deseeded and diced

3 spring onions, sliced

1 tablespoon sunflower oil

1 tablespoon hazelnut oil

1 tablespoon light soy sauce

1 clove garlic, crushed

Sea salt and ground black pepper

Directions

Cook the rice in a large pan of boiling water for about 30 minutes or until cooked. Drain well and cool. Put the cooled rice in to a large serving bowl and add the pineapple pieces (reserving the juice), sweetcorn, sultanas and red pepper and mix lightly. Make the dressing by taking the pineapple juice and combining with the soy sauce, oils and garlic. Season with salt and pepper. Mix well and pour over the salad. Garnish with the sliced spring onions.

8. **Salad nicoise**

Ingredients

225g new potatoes, small

225g tomatoes

200g fine green beans

4 handfuls of flat leaved parsley

4 spring onions

1 cos lettuce

1 red pepper

1/2 cucumber

115g of pitted black olives

200g tin tuna chunks in oil

100g anchovy fillets, drained, rinsed and chopped in half

3 eggs

Dressing:

3 tablespoons linseed oil

2 tablespoons olive oil

1 tablespoon balsamic vinegar

1 garlic clove, crushed

Sea salt and ground black pepper

Directions

Cook the green beans in boiling water for 2 minutes, drain and cool. Add the potatoes to boiling water and simmer until just tender. At the same time boil the eggs in a separate pan for 11 minutes. While these are cooking shred the lettuce leaves and place at the bottom of a large salad bowl. Chop the spring onions and sprinkle over the lettuce. Slice the cucumber lengthways and then in to small chunks. Deseed the pepper and cut in to thin strips. Add to the bowl. Drain the tuna and add half to the bowl together with half the anchovies and half the olives and half the parsley. Drain the eggs and immerse in cold water. Cut the potatoes in to chunks or halves and add to the bowl together with the green beans. Make the dressing by crushing the garlic and adding to the oils and balsamic vinegar. Add sea salt and black pepper to taste. Pour the dressing on to the salad and mix well. Shell the eggs and cut in to uarters. Add the remaining tuna. Arrange the eggs and the remaining olives, anchovies and parsley on top of the salad.

9. Tofu, noodle and sprouted bean salad

Ingredients

600g mixed sprouted beans and pulses (such as sprouted red lentil, mung, chickpea, aduki)

6 spring onions, shredded

2 large tomatoes, seeded and roughly chopped

1/2 cucumber, deseeded and diced

6 tablespoons fresh coriander

4 tablespoons fresh chopped mint

200g firm tofu, diced

50g vermicelli thread noodles

6 tablespoons rice vinegar

3 teaspoons caster sugar

3 teaspoons sesame oil

1 teaspoon chilli oil

Sea salt and ground black pepper

Directions

Pour boiling water over the thread noodles in a bowl and leave to soak for 3 or 4 minutes. Drain and run under cold water and drain again. Cut the noodles in to 2″ lengths and put in to a bowl. Put 500ml of water in to a wok or saucepan and bring to the boil. Add the beans and pulses and blanch for one minute, then drain. Add to the noodle bowl with the spring onions, tofu, tomato, cucumber and herbs. Make the dressing by combining the rice vinegar, sugar, sesame and chilli oils. Add to the noodle mixture and toss.

10. Baked stuffed aubergine

Ingredients

4 medium aubergines

1 red pepper, deseeded and chopped

1 yellow pepper, deseeded and chopped

1 green pepper, deseeded and chopped

1 large onion, chopped

2 cloves garlic, chopped

6 large ripe tomatoes, chopped

3 tbsp water

2 tbsp fresh parsley, chopped

Chopped mint and soya yoghurt to serve

Directions

Pre-heat the oven to 350C/180F/Gas 4.

Cut the aubergines in half lengthways and remove the flesh, retaining the skins intact. Heat the oil and cook the onion over a low heat until it starts to turn brown. Add the chopped peppers and the garlic and continue to cook for a further 5-7 minutes. Add the aubergine flesh and the tomatoes and simmer gently for 10 minutes. Add sea salt and pepper to taste and stir in the parsley.

Brush the aubergine skins with oil an place in a large roasting tin. Divide the filling between them. Drizzle a little more oil over the aubergines, put the water in the bottom of the roasting tin, cover with foil and bake for 40 mins until tender. Serve with the yoghurt mixed with the mint.

11. Mackerel and black beans

Ingredients

12 x 100g mackerel fillets

200g Portobello mushrooms

4 tbsp soy sauce

2 tbsp cooked black beans

2 tbsp olive oil

2 teaspoons sesame oil

3 garlic gloves, sliced thinly

8 spring onions, shredded, for garnish

Directions

Heat the oil in a saucepan. Grill the mackerel fillets for 2 minutes on each side. Meanwhile fry the garlic for 2 minutes. Add the soy sauce, black beans and mushrooms and cook for a further 3 minutes. Put the fish on a serving plate. Spoon the mushroom and black bean mixture over the fish. Garnish with the spring onions and lightly drizzle over the sesame oil.

12. Soy teriyaki salmon and noodles

Ingredients

500g skinless salmon fillet

300g dried egg noodles, cooked and drained

6 tbsp sweet sherry

3 tbsp olive oil

3 tbsp soy sauce

11/2 teaspoons soft brown sugar

75g alfalfa sprouts

50g sesame seeds

3 teaspoons grated fresh root ginger

2 cloves garlic, crushed

Directions

Slice the salmon thinly and soak for 40 minutes in the marinade of soy sauce, sherry, sugar, ginger and crushed garlic.

Drain the salmon and retain the marinade.

Heat the oil in a wok. Cook the salmon in the wok for 2 to 3 minutes and remove from the wok and keep warm. Add the marinade and noodles to the wok and stir fry for 4 minutes. Stir in the alfalfa sprouts. Transfer to serving plate and place the salmon on top. Sprinkle over the sesame seeds. Serve immediately.

13. Mushroom stroganoff with tofu

Ingredients

300g tofu, cut in to small cubes

2 onions, sliced

300g button mushrooms, sliced

300ml sour cream

4 tbsp olive oil

1 tbsp soy sauce

1 tbsp Worcestershire sauce

1 tbsp paprika

Lemon juice

Boiled brown rice

Directions

Marinate the tofu in the soy, Worcestershire sauce and half the paprika for 45 minutes. Heat just 2 tbsp of the olive oil in a frying pan and cook the onions with the paprika until the onions are translucent. Add the tofu and brown on both sides. Keep warm. Heat the remaining 2 tbsp of oil in the frying pan and fry the mushrooms for 2 minutes. Put all the ingredients back in to the frying pan, together with the sour cream. Mix well and bring back to a simmer for two minutes. Serve with brown rice.

14. Rich mung bean stew

Ingredients

300g mung beans, soaked overnight

4 tbsp tomato puree

2 tbsp olive oil

2 garlic cloves, crushed

1 onion, chopped

3 tbsp tomato puree

500ml red wine (optional)

1 green pepper, deseeded and diced

1 red pepper, deseeded and diced

1 fresh chilli, seeded and finely chopped

400ml water

Directions

Once soaked, put the mung beans in a large pan, cover with water and bring to the boil. When cooked, remove the saucepan from the heat. Drain and mash until smooth.

Heat the olive oil in a separate pan. Add the garlic and onion and fry for 5 minutes. Add the tomato puree and cook for 3 minutes, stirring well.

Stir in the mashed beans, then add the chopped peppers and chilli and red wine (if using). Add the water and stir well so that everything is mixed. Bring to the boil and simmer for 10 minutes. Serve straight away.

15. Salmon on lentils

Ingredients

6 salmon fillets

3 tablespoons toasted sesame seeds

2 tbsp olive oil,

6 shallots, finely chopped

2 carrots, finely grated

200g puy lentils

2 tbsp pine nuts

For the marinade:

2 tbsp olive oil

Freshly s ueezed lime juice

3 teaspoons soy sauce

2 tsp finely chopped root ginger

Directions

Mix the marinade ingredients together and add the salmon. Cover and leave for 1 hour turning the salmon after 30 minutes.

Cook the lentils. Heat the oil in a saucepan and fry the shallots until translucent. Add the carrots and lentils and stir well. Bring to the boil, cover and simmer for 40 minutes until lentils are soft. 10 minutes before the lentils are cooked, drain and dry the salmon. Grill or griddle for 4 minutes on each side. Heat the marinade and simmer for two minutes. Spoon the lentil mixture on to individual plates, put a salmon piece on top of each. Spoon a little marinade over each salmon piece and sprinkle with sesame seeds.

16. Butter bean, anchovy and coriander pate

Ingredients

800g (two large tins) butter beans, drained and rinsed

100g canned anchovy fillets in oil

5 spring onions, finely chopped

2 tbsp olive oil

3 tbsp lemon juice

6 tbsp fresh coriander, chopped

Salt and ground black pepper to taste

Lemon slices to garnish

Directions

Put the butter beans, anchovy fillets, spring onions, olive oil and lemon juice in to a blender with salt and ground pepper to taste. Blend to a coarse puree. Stir in the coriander. Garnish with lemon slices. Serve with toasted wholemeal bread.

17. **Butter bean, anchovy and coriander pate**

Ingredients

800g (two large tins) butter beans, drained and rinsed

100g canned anchovy fillets in oil

5 spring onions, finely chopped

2 tbsp olive oil

3 tbsp lemon juice

6 tbsp fresh coriander, chopped

Salt and ground black pepper to taste

Lemon slices to garnish

Directions

Put the butter beans, anchovy fillets, spring onions, olive oil and lemon juice in to a blender with salt and ground pepper to taste. Blend to a coarse puree. Stir in the coriander. Garnish with lemon slices. Serve with toasted wholemeal bread.

18. **Home made hummous with three seed biscuits**

Ingredients

800g (two large tins) of cooked chickpeas, drained

3 garlic cloves, chopped

90g pitted black olives

2 tbsp linseeds (flax)

150ml tahini paste

Juice of 2 lemons

2 tbsp extra virgin olive oil

1/2 pint water

Salt to taste

Few whole black olives, cayenne pepper and flat leaf parsley to garnish

Directions

Drain and rinse the chickpeas, cover with fresh cold water and bring to the boil in a saucepan. Boil rapidly for 5 minutes then reduce the heat and simmer gently for an hour or until soft. Put the chickpeas in a blender and process to a coarse puree. Add the linseeds, tahini paste, lemon juice, olive oil, black olives, 1/2 pint water and salt. Blend briefly. Transfer to a serving dish. Drizzle with a little olive oil. Sprinkle with cayenne pepper. Garnish with a couple of whole black olives and flat parsley leaves. Serve with warm pitta bread or three seed biscuits

19. Savoury three seed biscuits

Ingredients

300g wholemeal flour

6 tbsp sunflower oil

25g sesame seeds

25g linseeds

20g poppy seeds

1 tsp sea salt

1/2 tsp sodium bicarbonate

1 tbsp malt extract

Directions

Mix the seeds with the salt and sodium bicarbonate. Add the seeds, salt and sodium bicarbonate to the flour. Mix well. Mix the oil and malt extract. Gradually add the oil to the flour mixture to make a dough. Roll out the dough thinly on a lightly floured surface. Cut in to 3cm s uares or use a cookie cutter. Place on a lightly greased baking tray. Bake in a pre-heated oven at 350F/180C/Gas 4 for 10 minutes.

20. Sweet linseed and almond biscuits

Ingredients

200g wholemeal flour

200g soft brown sugar

200g chopped almonds

100g fine oatmeal or porridge oats

100g butter

250ml live yoghurt, preferably soya yoghurt

75g whole linseeds

50g fresh linseed meal

2 eggs

1 tsp vanilla essence

1 tsp baking powder

1/2 tsp sea salt

Directions

Soak the whole linseeds in the yoghurt. In a separate bowl, cream the butter, sugar, eggs and vanilla essence. Add the wholemeal flour the linseed meal, the oats, baking powder, sea salt and almonds, then combine with the yoghurt and whole linseed mix. Form in to balls. Place on a lightly greased baking sheet. Leave 5 cm between each ball. Cook in a pre-heated oven at 180C/350F/Gas 4 for 15 mins

21. Mixed seed and honey bars

Ingredients

100g sunflower seeds, lightly toasted

100g sesame seeds, lightly toasted

100g poppy seeds

100g linseeds

500g honey

2 tbsp lemon juice

1 tsp olive oil

Olive oil for greasing

Directions

Oil a shallow dish or swiss roll tin and set aside. Add the tsp of olive oil to a large saucepan and make sure that the inside is well coated. Put the lemon juice and honey in to the saucepan, mix well. Without stirring, bring to the boil over a medium heat. Once it is boiling, stir continuously until it reaches 140C/280F (test by dropping a little in to cold water. When ready it should turn in to hard but elastic strands). Take off the heat and stir in the seeds, then uickly pour in to the prepared dish or swiss roll tin. Cool for 10 minutes and then mark out in to about 12 bars, using a wetted knife. When completely cool, cut in to bars.

22. Summer pudding

Ingredients

Wholemeal bread, 6-8 thick slices

750g mixed berries (blackberries, blueberries, raspberries, redcurrants, strawberries)

50g stoned cherries

6 tablespoons honey

Soya yoghurt to serve

Directions

Cut the crusts off the bread and line the bottom and sides of a 850ml (11/2 pint) pudding basin making a good fit.

Put all the fruit and the honey in a large saucepan and cook for 4-5 minutes on a low heat. Stir carefully so as not to damage the shape of the berries. Remove from the heat and spoon the fruit and juices in to the lined pudding basin. Keep back 3 tablespoons of juice. Cover the fruit with more bread and place a plate slightly smaller than the basin on top of the pudding and weigh down with something like a large tin. Chill for a minimum of 4 hours. When ready to serve, turn the pudding out on to a serving plate. Trickle over the remaining juice. Serve with soya yoghurt.

Made in the USA
Las Vegas, NV
01 March 2024

86583759R00056